OFFICER DOWN

OFFICER DOWN

A Police Surgeon and the NYPD

FRANCIS V. ADAMS

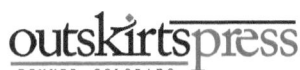
outskirtspress
DENVER, COLORADO

Also by Francis V. Adams:

The Asthma Sourcebook
The Breathing Disorders Sourcebook
Healing Through Empathy
Healing Through Empathy: An Expanded Edition

To the men and women of the NYPD who are truly New York's finest:
Be well and stay safe.

In memory of my friend, colleague, and honorary Police Surgeon Jacob
("Jack") Hirsch, M.D.
who suggested that I join the NYPD.

For LAA

Table of Contents

INTRODUCTION

I HAVE GOTTEN A NUMBER OF REACTIONS WHEN I TELL SOMEONE that I am a police surgeon with the NYPD. The most common is an inquisitive look of surprise. I may hear "I didn't know you operated" or "I didn't know you were a surgeon too." My friends and patients know me as an Internist who specializes in lung disease, so the "surgeon" job description always produces a reaction. The NYPD formed this medical unit of part--time doctors in the 1930s to manage the care of its members. The term is more commonly used in Europe, where it is synonymous with pathologists who practice forensic medicine. They perform autopsies and investigate crime scenes. *Police Surgeon* was also a short--lived television series in the UK in 1960 and featured Ian Hendry as Dr. Geoffrey Brent, a forensic pathologist. The show gets its notoriety from the fact that its creator, Sydney Newman, took Hendry and co--star Ingrid Hafner to a new series called *The Avengers* when *Police Surgeon* was cancelled after one season. *The Avengers* would become the longest running espionage series produced for English--language television.

It's largely the public's unfamiliarity with the term and what a police surgeon does that prompted me to write this book. In this country police surgeons come from a variety of medical specialties. The NYPD is based on the military model where rank is supreme and police surgeons hold the high rank of Inspector. By the nature of their work and the provisions of their labor contract, police officers have unlimited sick leave. A police surgeon became necessary to establish fitness for duty when a member of the service was absent due to illness. This was not only to ensure fitness, but also to identify malingering. Many of the injuries officers sustain are severe and complex, and a physician was deemed necessary to determine if care was being delivered properly. The Medical Division of the NYPD now has 31 physicians on staff as well as 300 "honorary," or voluntary, police surgeons who provide their expertise in every medical specialty.

The NYPD has divided the New York region into medical "districts" based on zip code. If an officer calls in sick he has 48 hours to return to duty. If not able to return the officer must report to his "district surgeon." Members of the service have health insurance and primary physicians so that the role of the surgeon is primarily one of review, rather than hands-on care. If a member of the NYPD is hospitalized, a police surgeon is dispatched to the hospital to assess the injury and the care that the officer is receiving. If the facility is unable to handle a severe injury, the surgeon will direct transfer to an appropriate center. Many of these "trauma calls" require police escort in the middle of the night, with sirens blaring and adrenalin rushing. A catastrophic event such as 9/11, a steam pipe explosion, or a crane collapse will bring an outpouring of officers into a hazardous environment. Here a police surgeon—or surgeons—will be on duty to oversee decontamination of civilians and officers and to triage injured personnel to area hospitals. I was on duty the night that a steam pipe exploded near Grand Central Station in Manhattan in 2007.

This book is about the men and woman of the NYPD, their injuries, and the role of a police surgeon in their recovery, as told through my experiences on the job. It is also about the impact of these experiences on my life. I joined the force at age 60 with nearly thirty years of experience in the practice of medicine but quickly found that I had to learn a new set of skills. I also had to adjust to the chain of command and a military--like organization. Each day on the force has brought a parade of officers into my district office with their injuries, some of which I may have already heard of that morning from reading my newspaper or listening to my car radio. I have met cops who have been portrayed in the media as heroes and as demons. My work as a police surgeon has brought excitement into my life at a time when many of my colleagues are retiring. It has also brought tough decisions. In many instances I have had to tell an officer that I believe that his injury prevents him from returning to work and that he should retire. At other times I've placed a member of the service back to duty when the officer believed that he was not ready. These decisions at times are met with resistance and anger.

The reader will meet officers who have been injured on the job and off, with minor and disabling injuries. In some cases these stories may reflect the dangerous nature of police work. In others, injury may have occurred by chance, off duty. In all instances the reader will see the interaction of the police surgeon with the member of the service and, at times, the department itself. It is my hope that this information will allow a view of the police department and of its members that has not been seen before.

Names, dates, places, and incidents in this book have been changed or omitted to ensure the security, safety, and wellbeing of the people, places, or agencies involved. Any resemblance to anyone living or dead is purely coincidental.

CHAPTER 1.

DUCHESS

I TOOK THE OATH OF POLICE SURGEON WITH THE NYPD DECEMBER 11, 2006, not entirely sure what my job would entail. I knew that any police officer who reported sick had to be seen by a police surgeon to ensure that he was receiving the proper care and to evaluate his fitness for duty. I also knew that I would be going to see any officer hospitalized during 12- to 24-hour shifts, in rotation with my fellow surgeons. At age 60, I wondered if I was too old or rigid to take on this position. After more than 30 years in the private practice of pulmonary and internal medicine I was quite comfortable as my own boss. I would now have to follow the chain of command and assume a supervisory role, rather than the "hands on" approach that I was accustomed to.

The department had recruited me with the prospect that I would be working on cases of officers injured on 9/11. Nearly ten years after the World Trade Center catastrophe, 9/11 respiratory issues remain a subject of daily concern to the general public, the medical community, and especially services like the NYPD and FDNY, with large numbers of members who were first responders to ground zero. There is also concern regarding future symptoms and the possible development of illnesses, including malignancy, in these groups. I had seen a small number of police officers and firemen with respiratory problems that had developed after 9/11 in my private practice, so the possibility of being involved in a larger number of cases provided me with motivation to join the NYPD. I also learned at my initial interview that I would be expected to man a medical district somewhere in the five boroughs where officers who had called in sick would report.

In order to learn the system and protocols I sat in with other police surgeons for several days and then started seeing officers individually in my assigned district, which turned out to be in the Bronx. I was immediately amazed by the litany of injuries these men and women had experienced. It seemed to me that every conceivable body part had been lacerated, fractured, sprained, strained, or operated on. With my own slipped disks, torn meniscus, arthroscopic surgery, torn rotator cuff, frozen shoulder, and four stints in physical therapy, my age and experiences as a patient proved to be an advantage. I had instant empathy with these resilient, but battered, men and women.

The first officer I saw was a young woman who entered the examination room wearing dark glasses. She had been qualifying at the firing range and a freak ricochet had pierced her eye, lacerating it nearly in half. Surgeons had sutured her globe and her vision had begun to return to normal. Despite her discomfort, she was anxious to return to work. A number of individuals entered the room on crutches or in braces, slings, or immobilizers. One young man was very somber; his eyes would not meet mine. A few days earlier he had discharged his weapon; a justifiable shooting, but with obvious lasting effects on his psyche. On a busy day I found myself seeing up to 35 officers who had reported sick. It did not take me long to observe that most police officers loved their job and, once injured, could not wait to get back to full duty.

A number of injuries involved dogs that had been trained by their criminal owners to attack. According to police guidelines, officers may not use deadly force against dogs except to protect themselves or others from physical injury, and there is no other means to eliminate the threat. In 2006 NYPD officers discharged their weapons 126 times and thirty times they fired at dogs. These encounters are especially difficult for those officers that love animals.

I recently met a Detective who was about to arrest a suspect when the perpetrator unleashed his German shepherd.

He described what happened."She was a beautiful dog, maybe 85 pounds and coming at me. I ran."

It surprised me that he had admiration for this animal, knowing how fierce the dog must have appeared.

"I was about to jump a fence when I felt her teeth breaking the skin of my thigh. I jerked away from that bite, but in a second I felt her teeth on my left arm. I had no choice. I pulled my gun and shot. I could see from her collar that her name was Duchess."

The Detective was overcome with guilt after the incident. I told him that I had just seen another officer whose arm had been badly broken by a dog in a similar situation and that I was sure there had been no alternative. Full of remorse, he decided to buy a dog and to give it the same name. By caring for this animal he would shed his guilt. I asked if it was another German shepherd.

"No," he said with a grin. "Duchess is a Yorkie."

CHAPTER 2.

NOT LIKELY[1]

POLICE SURGEONS IN EUROPEAN COUNTRIES ARE FORENSIC PATHOL-ogists who perform autopsies and investigate crime scenes. In this country, police surgeons are drawn from a variety of medical specialties and are responsible for the wellbeing of police officers. My weekday trauma call begins at 6PM and ends at 6AM the next morning, so whenever I awake at my usual time of 5:15 I immediately think that I am certain to get called. I always grab my cell phone on the way out to walk my dogs in case an officer is injured and a police surgeon is needed. I have been on the job for about ten months, so I am still relatively new to this position. Today the phone rang at 5:31 and I knew instinctively that it was the Sick Desk. The sergeant confirmed that I was on call and proceeded to tell me than an officer had been shot and had been taken to a local hospital. He said that the officer was "not likely."

What he meant was that the officer was not likely to die. I had heard this expression for the first time about a month ago, when I was asked to see an officer who had been severely injured in a motorcycle accident. "They say he's likely," the sergeant said. I paused, "Does that mean...?" "Right, he's likely," he repeated.

I asked for the specifics on today's incident; the officer's name, if he was still in the ER, or if he was in surgery. "We don't have much....no

---

1   Published May 5, 2008 "Police Surgeon and Officer Dodge A Bullet," Los Angeles Times

details….but he's in the ER." The sergeant said he was going to call the Chief Surgeon, and I told him that I would call in after I got to the hospital.

I knew it would take me at least 30 minutes to reach the hospital since I had been called there a few months ago to see an officer who had been attacked by a prisoner he was guarding. As I drove I thought about what I might encounter. In fact, I had thought about this happening for months. Shootings occur frequently, so that I knew it was inevitable that I would hear the words, "COP SHOT" on my watch. How would I handle it? The job of a police surgeon is to ensure that the member of the service is receiving the best possible care. I would have to quickly assess the medical condition of the injured officer as well as how the hospital was addressing his injuries. To do this I would need information from the physicians caring for him. On my last call I had no problem gathering information, but that had not been true for all of the hospitals I had visited.

From my previous calls I also knew that I would encounter a contingent of officers, both outside and within the hospital, and that the more serious the injury, the greater their number. I anticipated seeing patrol cars lined up outside of the ER. I was also certain to meet the officer's family at the bedside. Having watched the local news for many years, I expected that both the Police Commissioner and the Mayor would be there for a life threatening injury. My fellow police surgeons had told me that the Chief Surgeon would probably see any serious gunshot injury, in which case I might not be needed.

"How bad is this guy?" I thought.

I got the answer from my car radio. "A police officer was shot early this morning….." I turned up the volume. The officer was described as "lucky" by the reporter, who said that someone had fired on him from a rooftop and that the bullet had hit him in the arm. It was not a serious injury. I breathed a little easier as I drove. The officer would survive and so would I. My first shooting would be a minor wound. I thought about what I would say to the officer when I met him.

After about 35 minutes and one wrong turn I was within two blocks of the hospital when my car phone went off. It was the Sick Desk. "Dr.

Adams, what's your location?" "I'm just arriving at the hospital." The sergeant sounded disappointed. "I was hoping to catch you before you got there. The officer was not seriously wounded. It was a SCRATCH," he said emphatically. "The bullet just grazed him. He was released 10 minutes ago." A pause. "Oh and the Chief Surgeon got there and saw him. He appreciates your effort."

I made a left turn and headed toward my medical district where I would see officers who had reported sick. My role as police surgeon was becoming more familiar to me. With my long experience in practice I was comfortable dealing with illness, hospitals, and concerned friends and family, but I was not yet accustomed to violence and violent injuries. Today I was relieved that the officer was not seriously injured, but I also knew that one day I would be called for a more serious—even fatal—injury. Sadly, I know that call is coming. I know it's likely.

CHAPTER 3.

THE OFFICER WHO COULD NOT CROSS THE BRIDGE

I LIED TODAY. I LOOKED RIGHT INTO MY PATIENT'S EYES AND TOLD her something that was not true. I felt that I had no choice, but as a physician this is something that I have said I would never do. In thirty-plus years in practice, I have kept my word. Yes, I have omitted things or danced around the truth when a patient has told me that he does not want to know. Many people will tell me this in relation to cancer or a serious illness. "Don't tell me I have cancer or I'm going to die, I can't handle it." I might have to do the same thing with a critically ill, anxious patient, who I feel will decompensate with this information. In all of these circumstances I try to work with the patient's family as well as with the patient. In general I feel that the more the individual knows the better; but not today.

I was at my medical district, seeing members of the NYPD, as their police surgeon. Members of the service who are out sick must be seen to determine that they are receiving the proper care and to decide when they are able to return to work. Officers coming to their district surgeons are usually out of uniform, so many times I have trouble picturing the member of the service as a cop. The officer in front of me was one of those. She was a petite woman, between 100 and 110 pounds when I met her, with short dark hair. Size does not always equate with strength, but I wondered how this slight woman could subdue and arrest a violent criminal. The officer was articulate and mentioned that her role in the police department was to generate statistical reports. "I'm usually behind a desk," she told me.

I could see that she was distraught. "I'm not eating or sleeping and I've lost a few pounds. I'm afraid to go out and I think I have agoraphobia. I don't want to drive, I can't cross a bridge, and I don't want to see people."

She said she was staying in bed a lot and I commented that some of what she had described could be due to depression. I told her that she needed to see someone who was trained in that area and she agreed to be seen by one of the department's psychiatrists.

Before she left, she asked me if I had any experience with this type of disorder and I told her that I certainly had encountered these problems in my own practice and that depression had struck members of my own family. I told her that I thought it took courage to face this illness and to work with a psychiatrist to get better. I could tell from her expression that the personal reference had struck home. For a second I saw what was coming next and I regretted making that statement.

"The person in your family… How did that person do? What helped the most?" The officer was assuming that there had been a good outcome when, in fact, the person I was referring to had lost her life to depression. I could see that the officer was fragile, so I lied. I told her that with support, medication, and an interested physician, my family member had made it back.

Should I have told her the truth? I slept fitfully that night, uncomfortable with my decision, but certain that a truthful answer would have aggravated her depression. I resolved to tell her the truth if she recovered. I hoped that I would have that opportunity.

CHAPTER 4.

WOUNDS[2]

I EXPECTED TO SEE GUNSHOT WOUNDS WHEN I BECAME A POLICE surgeon. I had seen my first one as an intern decades earlier – a suspect injured during a robbery had been brought into the emergency room – and I still recalled the jagged, deep crater left by the bullet. The image had left its mark on me, not only by its appearance, but because it had been inflicted by another human being.

I was braced for the sight of other such disturbing wounds, but I was surprised to find that many injuries resulted from trips, stumbles and mishaps that occurred off duty. Among these were a detective who had grasped a glass that shattered, lacerating her hand and severing tendons and nerves supporting her thumb, and a sergeant building a deck on his home who had fallen through it, breaking several ribs. At first I thought this odd, that members of the police department, empowered by the law, would be as vulnerable as the rest of society.

But soon I was to learn that these men and women were vulnerable to dual risks: the ordinary dangers that all of us encounter from time to time – and the kind created by the violent society in which we live. And sometimes, I was to find, the most difficult--to--treat wounds weren't to the body.

2   Published November 23, 2009 "An NYPD Surgeon Learns the Random Nature of Wounds", Los Angeles Times

The first incident to drive this point home involved an officer who had been riding in a van with seven other members of the New York Police Department, about to be deployed for parade security. The van had stopped at a traffic light and the officer heard shouting. He saw a group of men and women standing on the sidewalk only a few feet away and a man nearby brandishing what appeared to be a handgun at them. Before the officer could react the gunman walked a few steps closer to the group on the sidewalk and fired, killing one of the men.

The officer later described the noise: "It was a .45, and it sounded like a cannon. I had never been that close to a gun firing without my ears being covered." The group in the van took cover, but the gunman had seen the NYPD logo and began to shoot. Three bullets struck the vehicle as the driver pulled away, stopping a half block up the street, where the officers disembarked, weapons drawn. No one inside the van had been hit, but at the street corner the gunman was still firing. Another man fell. The officer who had witnessed the first shooting returned fire with his colleagues, one of whom hit the gunman. In a few seconds, all shooting stopped.

The officer recounted: "My head was pounding and my ears were ringing. I could feel my heart beating. "

Sirens of other police vehicles and paramedics gradually became louder as the vehicles descended on the scene. All of the officers involved were taken to the nearest emergency room. Once released, they spent the remainder of the day and night answering questions regarding the shooting.

The officer whose head ached and ears rang was placed on medical leave and instructed to see his district police surgeon – me. Police surgeons supervise the care of injured officers and decide when they can return to duty, and I've found that it's impossible not to form relationships with these men and women.

In this case, the officer told me that in the 24 hours since the shooting his headache had become less severe. And although the ringing in his ears was softer, his hearing was off. He had been on the force for four years and had never previously fired his weapon in the line of duty. I arranged for him to have his hearing checked and asked him to come back in a week.

If his headaches were still a problem, I would refer him to a neurologist. When he returned, I could see from the seriousness of his expression that he was still disturbed by what had happened. The incident's impact had nothing to do with his physical complaints. "It happened so suddenly," he said. "I know that there are a lot of sick individuals out there."

He had been forced to confront both his vulnerability and a police officer's capability to inflict deadly force. This was a much different wound from what a bullet or knife would make and one with which I was not yet familiar. I knew that the officer would undergo counseling required by the department and return to work once this had been completed. His expression seemed to brighten as we talked about returning to duty. "I really want to get back to work," he said, and I sensed that resuming his routine would be the best therapy I could recommend. As for my role as a police surgeon, I was beginning to realize that I would need to deal with many types of injuries as well as the violence that produced them. I did not know which would be harder.

CHAPTER 5.

STEAM

THE CALL FROM THE SICK DESK CAME AROUND 7:30 PM. THE SERgeant wanted to know if I had heard about the steam pipe explosion in midtown. In fact, I had just received a call from a friend who wanted to know if I was alright. When I asked what she was referring to, she told me about the blast that had occurred about 6 PM at Lexington & 41st Street. I live about sixteen blocks from the site, but other than the sound of sirens—which are common in Manhattan—I had been unaware of the explosion. I had just turned on the TV and was listening to news reports of the explosion when the phone rang.

"They want a police surgeon down there. You are to report to the decontamination post at 44th & Lexington. The Chief Surgeon may already be there."

This was my night to be on Trauma Call and to see injured police officers, but I had not anticipated that I might be called for this type of duty. I knew from the reports that the streets would be clogged with traffic, so I asked for a patrol car to pick me up and take me over. Officer Garcia (name changed) of the Highway Patrol arrived about a half hour later and with the help of his siren, we made it through traffic. On the way over I wondered what injuries I might see and whether I was equipped to handle them. I remembered an earlier steam pipe explosion in the Gramercy

Park area many years ago, which had produced asbestos contamination. Asbestos is a carcinogen and it may produce scarring of the lungs, but those effects take years to develop. The heat from the steam, however, could burn the lining of the upper and lower respiratory areas and produce immediate respiratory collapse.

As we neared the explosion site I wondered if I was still in the same city. Midtown Manhattan had been transformed. I saw barricaded streets with dozens of police officers, some wearing masks, fire engines, ambulances and a variety of other vehicles. Officer Garcia snaked his way through the barricades and parked his patrol car about a block away from where I was to report. I exited the car and almost immediately ran into the Chief Surgeon, who was wearing a face mask.

"We have to set an example so put a mask on. The air sample results won't be ready until tomorrow so until then we have to take these precautions. It's good to have a pulmonologist here. I want you to join the decontamination post at 44th & Lexington. Keep me informed."

As I walked to the decontamination post I saw groups of firemen in full gear sitting on the ground. Walking down Lexington Avenue I could see towering spot lights that had been set up around the site of the explosion. It was a typical muggy July night, and the illumination revealed a smoky effect as steam rose from the crater. Grand Central Station sat unusually quiet to my right and I was immediately aware of the lack of pedestrian traffic in this normally congested area.

At 44th & Lexington the decontamination unit was roped off and I nearly joined the line of police officers, MTA workers, and civilians waiting to be washed down. These men and women had either been caught in the explosion or were first responders to the disaster. Mud and debris had rained down upon them. The officers performing the decontamination looked like alien creatures in their white-hooded hazmat suits and black masks with large eye holes. Each person stepped into a portable bathtub and was hosed down and scrubbed with soap, then stepped into a second bath for rinsing. Once rinsed, the soaked and dripping individuals entered a blue tent and changed into white hazmat suits and yellow boots, placing their clothing into large clear bags. Once changed, they were individually screened by two police EMTs, who took their blood pressures and oxygen measurements.

As I observed this process I saw one of the Deputy Chief Surgeons, in full uniform, interviewing the decontaminated individuals. The Deputy Chief was supervising the decontamination post and I went up to him when he finished and asked what he wanted me to do. He told me that there had been few injuries to the responders. One of the MTA bus drivers he had just spoken to was complaining of chest discomfort, so he was about to be transferred by ambulance to Bellevue Hospital. The Deputy Chief walked me through the decontamination process, which seemed to be going smoothly. I decided to stay with the EMTs as they screened the people exiting from the blue tent.

I saw about 50 decontaminated officers sitting casually on the sidewalk just beyond the decontamination tent. Most were drinking bottled water and every few minutes a pizza would appear and be quickly consumed. An MTA bus was brought in and many of the officers chose to sit in the air-conditioned bus rather than in the heavy July air.

I stood over the shoulder of one of the EMTs as they interviewed the freshly decontaminated officers and civilians. Almost all were in good humor, without physical complaints, but I noticed that few of them had slow pulses. Their rapid heart rates gave away their anxiety. Once the screening was completed they were urged to drink water and to secure their clothing and belongings with tape. Everything would be tested for asbestos and, if not contaminated, returned to them. Contaminated items would be disposed of.

I noticed a K--9 officer and his German shepherd partner appear at the end of the line for decontamination. They entered the bath together and, after a slight shudder as the cold spray was applied, the officer and his partner were calmly cleaned and rinsed. No distinction was made between animal and human.

I spoke to several officers from different units. There was relief that this was not a terrorist attack and that there hadn't been more injuries. I visualized lines of hundreds of people needing decontamination or medical attention. I was relieved too. None of the individuals I saw required my attention. I had been at the site for about three hours and wondered if this would be the only call for the night. When there were no more individuals in line for decontamination I began to walk towards my home, but before I reached it I received a call for the same sergeant at the Sick Desk. There were two injured officers who had been hospitalized and I needed to go see both. One had developed an asthma attack at the explosion site and had been taken by ambulance to St. Vincent's Hospital. The second officer had had chest pains unrelated to the explosion and was at St. Luke's Hospital. These types of calls I was used to. I knew what I would be dealing with.

I told the sergeant that I would call in after seeing these officers and asked for Highway Patrol to pick me up again. I saw both officers, called in their status, and got home about 1:30 AM. Assuming that there would be no further calls I would have less than five hours of sleep before starting out in the morning, but even five minutes would have been welcome. There were no dreams that night, just dead out sleep. I slept knowing that I had not contributed much to tonight's effort but that I would be better prepared if something similar happened. I was certain that someday it would.

CHAPTER 6.

RMPs

RADIO MOBILE PATROL VEHICLES, OR RMPS, ARE POLICE CARS. I wasn't familiar with this term when I became a police surgeon. Cops speak a language of their own. I became aware of this as soon as I started listening to officers describing their injuries.

"I was responding to a 10--13 when my RMP was T--boned by another vehicle."

The officer had heard the radio signal for "officer needs assistance" while patrolling in his car and was struck from the side by another automobile. He had been taken to a nearby emergency room with complaints of neck, shoulder, and back pain. X--rays were negative for fractures, but he was still in considerable pain when he reported to the district the next day. "I can't lift my shoulder above here," he said (he had raised it to near shoulder level). I did a brief exam and concluded that he was badly bruised. "I'm going to authorize you to see an orthopedic specialist so we can be sure there is no tendon damage," I told him. When an officer is injured in the line of duty the police surgeon is the one who directs his care by authorizing consultations, tests, and treatment. Payment to treating physicians is through Workman's Compensation.

My officer saw an orthopedic surgeon who requested a shoulder MRI, which I approved. The MRI revealed a torn rotator cuff and the orthopedist requested approval to perform arthroscopic surgery. Requests for surgery require approval from the Medical Division's orthopedic surgeons and I referred my officer to see one our supervising surgeons. If approved, the officer would have the surgery and return to me periodically for monitoring of his recovery. I would place him back to duty, either "light" (desk work) or "full," when I felt that he was sufficiently recovered.

Almost every conceivable bone or joint may be injured in an RMP accident. Police vehicles often travel at high speeds. Many of the injuries that I have seen have occurred while officers were in pursuit or in transit to crime scenes. I have seen officers with fractures that I had never heard of and with torn tendons and ligaments that I had to look up in my old anatomy texts. On busy days at the district it would seem like I was seeing an endless array of large and small bumps, strains, sprains, fractures, and bruises.

At times RMP collisions may be violent. One officer showed me her totaled vehicle in a photo on her cell phone. "It took the FDNY a half hour to cut me out of there." Her injuries appeared minor in comparison to the wreck in the photo. I advised her to see an orthopedist to be sure that the ER and I had not missed anything. I asked her who she had collided with. "It was another RMP. We both were responding to the same call."

RMP accidents have increased in the last few years and this has attracted attention from the media and the Department. On average, 30 to 40 percent of all police pursuits nationally involve some type of accident. The NYPD has a strict policy on high-speed pursuits. Officers are instructed to follow a violent suspect who flees, not chase. They are also to avoid speeding through lights.

Accidents often occur after midnight. I was called out in the early morning on one of my first trauma calls to see two officers who had been involved in an RMP accident in Manhattan. They were still in the ER when I arrived and I found both men in a large, brightly lit cubicle. They were still awaiting x-- rays and CT scans to rule out spinal injuries. Both were immobilized on boards with neck braces, in case of cord injury. I learned that they had been travelling at a high rate of speed and were struck by another vehicle as they crossed an intersection. I introduced myself and asked the driver, Officer Murphy (name changed), how he was feeling. "Not bad. I have a headache. I'll be happy when I can move around." His partner was equally stoical. I spoke to the Attending Physician in the ER who said that their examinations did not reveal any neurological damage, but that he still wanted to get CT scans. Fortunately the scans were negative and both men were released several hours later.

An off-duty highway patrolman was not so lucky. He had been riding his motorcycle in Manhattan and collided with a speeding vehicle. The call from the Sick Desk informed me that he was "likely," meaning that he was not expected to live. I rushed to the ER to find Officer Perez (name changed) surrounded by several officers from his precinct and his wife. He had multiple fractures, including his ribs and legs, and there was some concern about a tear in his spleen. I spoke to the orthopedic resident who was about to take the officer to the OR to repair the leg fractures. Fortunately Officer Perez had been taken to one of the City's major trauma centers, so I felt confident he was going to receive the best possible care. I had been informed that the chairman of the orthopedics department at the hospital was an Honorary Police Surgeon and I made sure that he would be called. The officer made it through surgery, but due to the extent of his injuries he never returned to full duty and was retired.

It was only a few weeks later that I was called out for another motorcycle accident. A drunk driver had struck an off-duty officer. Again the injuries were extensive, but the officer survived. I met his wife outside his ICU cubicle and asked how she was doing. "I don't know. He's had so many dangerous assignments and come through without injury. Today he went out to get a quart of milk and he was almost killed." I had begun to appreciate what she was referring to. Many of the members of the service I had seen had been involved in high-risk situations prior to their injuries and had come through without injury. A few had been in Iraq as well, and had returned to begin or resume careers with the NYPD. I wondered if surviving these encounters unscathed created a false sense of security. I later learned that the injured officer recovered and was able to resume full duty with the NYPD.

Highway patrol (usually called "Highway") escorts police surgeons on trauma call to the hospital where an injured officer has been admitted. As I entered one RMP the officer asked me if "we were in a hurry?" I said yes, since I had been told that a sergeant on the force had been hospitalized with chest pains and a possible heart attack. With lights flashing we left and proceeded at high speed to our destination. Highway deftly zipped in and out of traffic, at times going up the wrong side of the street, and cleared our path of slowly moving vehicles with a variety of lights and sirens. Inside the RMP I noticed that the officer had to take one hand off the wheel in order to work these controls. I also eyed the speedometer as it hit 90 mph. During the entire trip I was sure we were going to be involved in an RMP accident. I wondered if another surgeon would have to be dispatched to see me. We made it to our destination without incident. My legs were a little rubbery as we exited the RMP and my pulse was racing. I saw the injured officer who had been admitted and found that the initial tests for a heart attack were negative. He would be admitted for observation. On the trip home I told Highway I wasn't in a hurry.

CHAPTER 7.

COPS ALL

ANY OFFICER, REGARDLESS OF RANK, WHO REPORTS SICK AND who cannot return to duty in 48 hours must be seen by his District Surgeon. This means that high ranking Inspectors and Captains may report to me along with police officers, sergeants, detectives, and lieutenants. I will also see injured cadets from the Police Academy. This has given me contact with a good cross section of the brass, as well as the rank and file of the Department. As in the military, rank matters. High-ranking officers are seen first, but report sick less often. Their injuries, however, are not much different from the rank and file, whether incurred on duty or off. One Inspector saw me for a few months after undergoing a total knee replacement. After he left my office on one visit the next officer in said he used to work with him. "You know he's a legend in the Department, don't you?" I said no and asked him to tell me why. The officer went on to describe how the Inspector had once taken on a gang of motorcycle thugs who were menacing the patrons of a bar. I wondered if that was how he had originally injured his knee. The Inspector did not stay out of work very long and requested to be put back to work as soon as he had finished rehabilitation.

Police officers come in all shapes and sizes. A number have entered my office who I swore could not be on the force. Unlike the FDNY, which insists on a yearly physical examination, the NYPD does not require regular examinations of its members. It is not unusual for me to see overweight officers. These same individuals might be diabetic or have heart disease or high blood pressure. Two officers in my district had undergone bariatric surgery for morbid obesity. On average, police officers exercise and remain in shape since they must be physically fit to perform their duties. A number of injuries that I have seen have occurred during foot pursuits where officers leapt and jumped fences or other objects attempting to apprehend suspects. One young officer reported to me after fainting on the job. He told me that in the heat of the summer he had been performing "a vertical." What he meant was that he had been assigned to patrol a high-rise building from lobby to roof, via the stairwells. After climbing several flights of stairs he had passed out and been taken to an ER. The ER examination showed that he was dehydrated and he was given IV fluids. By the time he reported to me he was feeling well and was anxious to return to duty. I advised him to stay well hydrated during the summer months, especially if he had to exert himself.

Women entered the NYPD in 1891. There are now over 3000 female officers in the NYPD, but few of high rank. These women perform the same duties as their male counterparts and experience similar injuries. I have seen a number that were injured grappling with suspects both male and female. Female officers have the same medical needs and problems as the civilian population so that it is not unusual for me to see an officer who is pregnant or who has undergone gynecological or cosmetic surgery. A young female officer saw me after injuring her knee in the line of duty. It was on her very first tour after graduating from the Academy and being assigned to a command. "I can't believe it happened on my first shift. I will never live this down." I had heard from other officers that new cops are often subject to razzing. I was sure that she did not want to appear to be weak in the eyes of her fellow officers. She asked to be put back to work as soon as possible.

I have seen two officers who were accused of being bad cops. The first was one of four officers indicted in a shooting. The other had been indicted for shooting a civilian while off duty during an altercation out-side of a bar. I tried not to judge these men; the courts had or would do so. I know that both of these officers appeared to have the weight of the world on their shoulders and felt pursued by the media. One described the press camped out in front of his home. At the time that they were seen they were both facing the possibility of conviction and incarceration. My impression was that both men had felt threatened and made split-second decisions to use deadly force.

Cops in general are young, upbeat, and love their work. They talk freely about "doing their twenty" (police officers have the option to retire after twenty years of service at 50 percent of their salary). Many stay on after twenty years, if they are physically capable. They are loyal to a fault, especially to their partners. Whenever I have visited a hospitalized officer there has been at least one member of the force at his bedside.

Sometimes the partner is an animal. One of my injured cops was with the K-9 unit. His partner, Max, a German shepherd, lived with him and his family. When the officer was out sick the dog stayed home as well. I asked how the family was getting along. "Max was not a family dog when I was working, but since I've been out he is not as high strung as he was. You'll find him sleeping on the sofa instead of patrolling the backyard. I'm wondering how he will be when we go back to work." The officer had worked with a human partner before joining the K-9 unit. I asked him who he preferred to work with. He did not hesitate to answer: "The dog." Several of my cops were with the mounted police, and they would all visit their horses when they were out sick. I could tell that they really missed their partners. One officer had been with the unit for nearly his entire career, just short of twenty years. Unfortunately it had taken its toll on his neck and back and he was forced to retire.

During my orientation I had been warned that I might face anger or even a lawsuit from officers who disagreed with my assessment of their fitness for duty. To date I have been always been treated with respect by the members of the service, even when I have returned officers to work who felt they were not ready. The vast majority of the officers I have seen have been anxious to get back to work. There are exceptions; I have seen members of the service who had been out of work or on desk duty for years after an injury. I have suggested to a number of officers who I felt could not return to full duty that they retire. This is always difficult since the average police officer assumes that he will complete his "twenty" without physical injury. Many love their work and are deeply disappointed that they cannot continue their career. I've also seen officers return to full duty with residual pain from their injuries. A few of these officers were unable to cope and ultimately retired.

When I see an officer who is about to retire I always ask what comes next. I had assumed that since most are relatively young they would all have a second career in mind. Many have had definite plans, but a number of the officers I have spoken to were unsure of the future. A detective in my district had to retire due to a severe shoulder injury. He had undergone three operations, hoping to be able to return to full duty, but unfortunately remained in severe pain. He was one of several officers I have met who had done a tour of duty in Iraq. Now that he was forced to retire he said he would try to get hired to teach at the Police Academy; something he had always wanted to do. I heard from him a few months after he left the force and he had not gone ahead with this plan due to persistent pain. He said he was still planning to teach. I wished him luck and hoped that he would have the chance to pursue his dream.

CHAPTER 8.

SHOT!

I'VE SEEN SEVERAL OFFICERS WHO HAVE BEEN WOUNDED IN THE line of duty, but I still have no idea of what it is like to be shot. I can imagine the horror of realizing that this is about to happen and I can certainly recall the worst pain I have ever felt and suspect that this is what it feels like, but I am still at a loss. I've read articles in which the wounded person is quoted as saying that he didn't know he had been shot or that only after a while did he realize what had happened. I've concluded that this relates to where the bullet enters the body and what it encounters.

A female undercover attempting to arrest an individual who was riding between subway cars in Brooklyn was shot in the leg, arm, and chest, after the suspect pulled a gun. The gunshot to her leg proved to be from friendly fire as two other officers fired upon the suspect who had grabbed the female officer in a headlock and pulled a 9mm handgun. I saw the officer in my district several weeks after she had been wounded. She was wheeled into my office by a member of her squad. Surgery had been performed on her leg and she was now in rehab. I found the officer to be in good spirits, but she still was experiencing significant pain. She was a ten-year veteran of the force who had planned to "do her twenty" until the shooting took place, but now had to face disability and retirement.

A detective in my district exchanged gunfire with a robbery suspect in

Manhattan and was shot in the ankle, shattering bone. The first time I saw him he was unable to climb the stairs to the second floor clinic so I came down to the first floor to see him. He was one of the officers I met who I had read about in the *Daily News* before meeting them in person. On his first visit his foot was still in a cast and he was requiring pain medication regularly. With each subsequent visit he seemed to shed various parts of the hardware needed to mend or support his ankle. Finally he walked into my office using a cane. Unfortunately he was in continuous pain and had lost feeling in his injured foot. The bullet had damaged a nerve that travels down the ankle to the foot. This proved to be a permanent injury and the detective was forced to retire.

I've also seen an officer who discharged his weapon by accident and shot himself in the foot. The wound was large and it had required surgery and further care when it became infected. I tried to read the officer's face as to how he felt about the situation, imaging considerable embarrassment, but I did not detect much more than the fact that he seemed calm and anxious to return to work. I put him back after several weeks, but I was not sure if he faced any departmental review of the shooting.

I was handed the chart not long ago of an officer and told by the clinic staff that "he comes in every six months." The NYPD will keep officers with severe line of duty injuries on active but "out sick" status indefinitely, so that they may receive their full benefits. I glanced at the chart and noticed that the officer had been shot eleven years ago. I asked him what had happened. He told me that he had been shot in the head and pointed to his left temple. "The bullet entered here and exited here (pointing to behind his right ear). It tore through my right eye and I'm legally blind in my left eye, which was hit too. They also had to remove part of my brain." I told him that from what I could see he had made an amazing recovery and he said that at the time he had not been expected to live. Except for his vision he seemed otherwise intact. He said that his fellow officers continued to help and that one had driven him to this appointment. I said, "From what I've seen the NYPD does take care of its own." He replied, "I'm living proof."

I've thought a lot about these officers that have been wounded on and off the job. I've gotten the impression that although they live with the possibility of serious injury every day, none of them expected that they would ever face a potentially fatal wound. Once wounded, all of these members of the force realized how vulnerable they were. In some instances their injuries were career--ending, while in others they were badges of honor. In all, the wounds proved to be life--altering and, for me, a sobering reminder as to how dangerous it is to be a police officer. In 2008, 133 police officers in this country were killed in the line of duty. Four were members of the NYPD.

CHAPTER 9.

WORLD TRADE CENTER

I WAS NOT YET A MEMBER OF THE NYPD ON SEPTEMBER 11, 2001 BUT it was the World Trade Center disaster that provided the impetus for me to join the force. As a lung specialist I was interested in the illnesses that had resulted from the inhalation of dust at ground zero, and in the years after 9/11 I had seen a few members of the NYPD and the FDNY in my private practice with respiratory problems. Like so many others I also wanted to make a contribution to the services that protect and rescue us. By the time I joined the force in 2006 several scientific reports of WTC--related illnesses among first responders had already been published.

The most common respiratory illness resulting from the collapse of the towers is termed "World Trade Center Cough Syndrome." This illness is the result of irritation to the nose, sinuses, throat, bronchial tubes, and esophagus of individuals exposed to WTC dust and fumes. The syndrome includes symptoms of rhino sinusitis, esophageal reflux, and asthma, often in combination. Less frequent respiratory illnesses attributed to ground zero exposure include sarcoidosis, an inflammatory illness of the lungs, and scarring or pulmonary fibrosis.

I saw my first case of WTC Cough Syndrome in a police officer in 2002. When I first met Jason Mendez (name changed) it wasn't his weight-lifter's biceps that impressed me — it was his formidable cough. Just as

Jason began to describe his illness he broke into a fitful bout of coughing and was unable to speak. Several bouts of coughing followed. During these paroxysms Jason turned red in the face and had trouble breathing. His chest heaved and his whole body convulsed as the fits of coughing continued. Jason told me that he had even passed out once after a severe attack.

I quickly recorded his history, which was that he had had no health or respiratory problems prior to 9/11 and that he was a first responder, arriving shortly after the first tower fell. I asked Jason if he had worn a mask and he said that none were available for the first few hours he had been on the pile. Later that day he was given a thin, carpenter--type facemask but it was only after almost 48 hours at ground zero that he received a mask with a built-in protective HEPA filter.

Jason started coughing on the evening of 9/11 and he continued to cough for more than a year, right up to our visit. His physical exam revealed inflammation of the nasal/sinus passages, and throat, as well as wheezing. I obtained a chest x--ray and breathing tests and concluded that the officer had asthmatic bronchitis, a condition in which the air passages of the lung are inflamed, narrowed, and irritable, mimicking asthma. I felt that the source was his WTC exposure. There was also evidence of nasal and sinus inflammation, indicative of rhino sinusitis. Jason's breathing capacity was only 60 percent of what was predicted for his age, weight, and sex. This was especially striking since he had never smoked and had been in excellent health prior to 9/11.

I obtained a CT scan of Jason's lungs, which showed that his bronchial tubes were thickened — a sign of bronchitis. There was no evidence of scarring on his lungs. An ear, nose, and throat physician performed an examination, which showed that Jason also had reflux of gastric contents into his esophagus. This condition may produce or exacerbate cough. The officer was treated with high doses of corticosteroids to reduce the inflammation of his airways, bronchodilators to open the passageways, and medication that reduces acid production in the stomach to reduce reflux. Jason's cough gradually subsided over several days and he was discharged.

I have followed Jason since 2002 and he remains on daily medication to control his condition. The officer still coughs and notes shortness of breath on exertion, but is able to lead an active life. He is one of several patients I have seen with WTC Cough Syndrome. The officer's cough has flared a few times since his initial presentation and each time I have treated him with short courses of steroids to bring it under control. His lung capacity has remained reduced despite treatment.

The long-term effects of pollutants released on 9/11 are still unknown. It is estimated that 525,000 people, including 90,000 workers, were exposed to toxic materials during the collapse, recovery, and cleanup efforts. When I speak to officers who were at ground zero they frequently express concern about the future and whether other diseases, especially cancer, might develop. The Department monitors its members for any unusual illnesses and 9/11 medical facilities continue to perform periodic examinations. I find that it is the uncertainty of what the future holds that most disturbs the officers I have met. During Jason's last office visit I reminded him of how sick he had been — that he could barely get a word out without coughing. He replied, "I know I'm a lot better, but it looks like I will never get rid of this cough. Can you tell me what comes next?" I had no answer and said, "We can only wait and see."

CHAPTER 10.

DOES ANYONE COME PEACEFULLY?

AFTER LISTENING TO OFFICERS DESCRIBE INJURIES INCURRED while arresting and subduing perpetrators I have often asked "Does anyone come peacefully?" The answer has always been "No."

It seems that suspects about to be placed under arrest are more likely to resist than surrender. The resistance is typically sudden and violent. Perpetrators caught in the act will often attempt to flee the scene, resulting in a chase or collision that is likely to produce injury. One officer described a violent encounter and said that he thought that his young suspect was out to prove himself. "I guess he saw an old man and thought he was stronger." As he spoke I noticed that the officer was graying at the temples and I wondered if the suspect had seen it too.

In some cases the suspect may be an "EDP" or "Emotionally Disturbed Person," a term the NYPD uses. These individuals may be intoxicated or mentally ill. One of the most common intoxications the officers I spoke to encountered was with methamphetamine, a powerful stimulant, which may produce agitation and aggression. In a number of instances the officers described how it took several men to subdue a suspect high on meth. Many times I have seen more than one of the arresting officers from the same incident and heard each one describe how they were injured. "I had his right arm and my partner had his leg. I got thrown to the floor and landed on my knee." While listening I try to visualize these altercations from the differing viewpoints and how these injuries occurred.

A number of hand injuries that I have seen have resulted from the handcuffing of suspects. I had thought of this as a simple procedure from watching TV shows and movies in which suspects willingly followed the direction to place each hand behind their back. I now know this to be a difficult and potentially dangerous maneuver, particularly when a suspect is resisting and uncooperative. Fingers, particular thumbs, may be caught in the clasp of the cuff or between metal and flesh, resulting in lacerations, fractures, or painful dislocations. The delicate network of nerves and tendons of the hand is often disrupted by these injuries — in some cases resulting in permanent disability. Sometimes the handcuff may even become a weapon. One officer described how he was lulled into a false sense of security when a perpetrator willingly allowed one hand to be cuffed and then suddenly ripped that hand away, striking the officer in the head with the dangling cuff. The officer, stunned and bleeding, fought back to subdue his suspect.

Hand-to-hand combat is not unusual in these violent altercations that occur daily. Listening to the descriptions of these events I often think of the men and women of the NYPD as modern day gladiators fighting for their lives, many times with only their hands and fists. The suspects, desperate to get away, are not hesitant to use any means to avoid arrest so it is not unusual for me to see an officer who has been punched, kicked, or bitten while attempting to apprehend an individual.

These often bloody confrontations may result in the exposure of the arresting officer to infectious diseases, particularly HIV. In these instances the officer may be judged at risk of infection and placed on prophylactic medication by an emergency room physician. This consists of the "HIV cocktail," which includes several antiviral medications. My role in these cases is to authorize serial blood tests for HIV and hepatitis, as well as consult with an Infectious Disease specialist. In most cases the member of the service will remain on the cocktail for thirty days to reduce the risk of HIV infection.

An undercover officer who attempted to arrest an individual he had observed dealing drugs reported to me with a splint on his right hand and bruises on his face and limbs. I asked him to tell me what had happened. "It all went down very quickly. He ran when I approached him. I chased him for several blocks and I went over a fence and bushes. Then I caught him. I know we were grappling on the ground. Punches were flying and there was blood; my hand, his face. In the ER they stitched the cut on my hand and said that his blood may have mixed with mine. They started me on the HIV medicine. I've only taken two doses and I've vomited and have diarrhea." I told him that these were common side effects of the HIV drugs and that they might last the full time he was on the medication. I authorized the necessary follow up for the body fluid exposure as well as an orthopedic consultation for his hand and told him it might be a tough month.

"But you got the guy," I said. The undercover grinned through his bruises and said, "Yeah, he's off the street for a while, maybe a long time." Then he added, "I'd do it all again."

CHAPTER 11.

THE 50ᵗʰ PRECINCT

MY ASSIGNED MEDICAL DISTRICT OFFICES ARE HOUSED ON THE second floor of the 50ᵗʰ Precinct, which is located in the Kingsbridge section of the North West Bronx. I was not familiar with this area prior to joining the NYPD but quickly discovered that the Precinct included Van Cortland Park, one of New York's largest, and bordered on the Hudson River. The area immediately surrounding the Precinct has a mix of residential and commercial areas and includes an elevated subway line. Just a few blocks from the Precinct is the factory that produces the Stella D'Oro brand products. This accounts for the enticing smell of fresh baked goods that I encounter frequently in my comings and goings to the district.

Unfortunately, that sweet oven smell is replaced by ones that are not as inviting, once you enter the station house, an uninviting structure on Kingsbridge Avenue. On most days you are met by the strong smell of antiseptic. My only previous visit to a police station was many years ago after my car had been stolen, so I had little to compare the 50ᵗʰ to when I arrived for duty. Station houses have often been depicted on TV and in the movies, however, and I found the precinct to resemble what I had seen in the media. The station house is a three-story brick structure and the décor is pure cinderblock, painted various colors. It is brightly lit, which serves to highlight its starkness. On entering, I noticed the sergeant sitting behind a long bench, which I took to be the booking area. I could see the entrance to holding cells off to the right and a large room where I assumed roll call took place was on the left. Police stations are not for comfort and the first summer I worked at the 50th was sweltering. Fortunately the next two years saw the addition of air conditioning. In the winter the station house is overheated, so that I found myself missing the summer months.

It is not unusual for me to see handcuffed suspects being booked as I enter and leave the station house. The arresting officers usually have one hand on the suspect's arm as they are lead up to the sergeant on duty and booked. Although I try not to, I find that I can't avoid looking at the faces of those who have been arrested. For most, there is a look of sad resignation or a blank stare. For the officers it appears to be business as usual, but I feel I can detect an air of self-satisfaction that they got their man.

The medical district offices are one flight up on the second floor. There is a waiting area that seats about 30 members of the service so that on a busy day, when more than one surgeon is present, officers will spill out to the hallway. The medical division sergeant and administrative assistants occupy one large room and the district surgeons and nurse are housed in small offices. The offices have blood pressure cuffs, otoscopes, ophthalmoscopes for looking in the eyes and ears, and exam tables, but they do not have sinks, so I doubt they were originally intended for medical use.

During my first year at the 50th Precinct the elevator was often out of service so that I had to go downstairs to see officers who had reported sick and were unable to climb the stairs. The large roll call room served as a temporary office. On one of these occasions I met a detective I recognized from reading my morning paper. He had been shot in the leg apprehending a robbery suspect in Brooklyn a few days before. The bullet had shattered several bones in his ankle and he had undergone surgery. He seemed anxious to talk about his injury. "They showed me the x--rays after they operated. I wanted to count the screws they put in, but there were too many." I asked him about the pain and he seemed to shrug it off. Like many other injured officers he said that he didn't like taking pain medication. "That stuff messes me up." I told him I had read that he had chased and caught the suspect after running several blocks, despite being wounded. "I don't know how you ran on that ankle. You're a hero," I said. The detective shrugged this off too. Then he said what was really on his mind. "I just want to walk again."

CHAPTER 12.

GUNS

NYPD OFFICERS CHOOSE FROM A LIST OF APPROVED ON AND OFF duty firearms. On duty, uniformed officers carry the Glock 26, Smith and Wesson 5946, or Sig Sauer 226 models. The members of the service may carry one of these firearms off duty, or select another, smaller weapon from an approved list. I've gotten used to the presence of firearms since officers may come into the medical district in uniform. Police surgeons are considered uniformed officers by the NYPD so that we may carry firearms. A few of my colleagues have qualified and "carry."

An officer's weapon is his lifeline and it must be secure and functional at all times. When an officer is injured or on medication, a police surgeon must determine if these conditions are still met. Removing a weapon from a member of the service, even temporarily, can be a difficult decision. At other times both the officer and surgeon recognize that it has to be done.

I had seen a young officer several times for a shoulder injury that had required surgery a few years ago. A recent RMP accident had aggravated the old injury and required physical therapy. After several weeks I returned the officer to full duty. Several months later he reported sick to the district, complaining of increased pain. I recognized the officer and asked him how he had been and he said, "Not great. I've got this bum shoulder and there are problems at home." I focused on his injury and authorized him to see his orthopedist for evaluation. The officer returned to me about a week later with a note from his physician stating that the injury was a minor sprain. I suggested that the officer return to work and he replied that he couldn't. "I've got too many problems. I'm not ready to go back. Can't you keep me out?" I asked him if it was his pain or other problems that prevented him from working and he did not answer. "Are you depressed?" I said and he replied, "I'm not sure." I wasn't certain if the officer was suffering from depression, but his frank reply left me convinced that I had to find out. There is a psychiatrist assigned to medical headquarters in Queens. "I'm going to send you right over to see the department's psychiatrist." The officer did not protest.

I saw him one more time in the district. He said he was receiving psychotherapy and taking antidepressant medication but wasn't feeling much better. "They say I don't have to come here anymore since my shoulder isn't the problem. I'm being followed by the department shrink. You're off the hook." He continued. "You know the day I was here a Detective came to my home to collect my weapons. I'm glad they're gone." The officer and I had come to the same conclusion.

CHAPTER 13.

A BAD YEAR

OFFICER WILLIAMS (NAME CHANGED) HAD HAD A BAD YEAR—OR at least that was how he put it when he sat down in my district office. "Out of all of these men, you are going to know my name by heart." He was right—I did know his name. I was seeing him for his fourth line of duty injury in a period of seven months. In fact, I had just put him back to work less than three weeks prior to this visit.

One of the reasons I remembered this particular officer was the violent nature of his last injury. When I hear about a particularly violent incident it will often stay in my mind—I try to visualize what happened. Officer Williams had been pursuing a robbery suspect on foot and caught his man. A struggle followed in which he was dazed and knocked to the ground. The suspect then proceeded to pound Officer Williams' head against the pavement several times. When he first told me this, I winced. "It's a good thing I have a hard head," he said. In the emergency room he described how the doctor in the ER removed road debris from his head wounds. When I saw him the next day his wounds were still weeping plasma. "I have a terrible headache," he said. "They said it's a concussion." I asked where his assignment was and he said that he patrolled housing in one of the most criminally active areas of the city. I authorized a consultation with a neurologist and the officer returned after two weeks, feeling better. "The doc says I'm okay. No brain damage," he smirked. His wounds were dry and his headaches had resolved. I returned him to full duty; but here he was in my office less than a month later.

"Tell me what happened," I said. Officer Williams said that he and his partner had observed a drug buy and were attempting to arrest the dealer, who resisted. "The perp and I were fighting and I was trying to get the cuffs on. My partner was trying to help, but the clasp of the cuffs punctured my hand. It went right through the skin below my thumb." In the struggle the three men had fallen in a heap and Officer Williams had emerged with a bleeding hand and soreness of his neck, shoulders, and back. He had been seen in an emergency room and released. "I'm pretty banged up. They say nothing's broken, though." I did a quick exam of the bruised areas and he was right, no fractures or dislocations. His hand had a puncture wound, which would heal without sutures.

I noticed that Officer Williams was not a big man. He was about 5 foot 8 inches tall, at best, and he was thin with a wiry frame. There was no bulk to him, unlike a lot of his fellow officers who did weight training. I know that size is not always equal to strength, but I wondered if he could be overmatched on the street. Did criminals size him up and think that he could be taken? I knew that his wounds would heal but I was concerned about what would happen next. "You've had a string of injuries this year," I said. "Yeah, I've had some run--ins. That first one I saw you for was my left arm and shoulder. That perp had me in a hold and twisted my arm and dislocated my shoulder. The next time was that shooting in the hallway of the high rise where I was doing a vertical. A gun went off right near my head and I had ringing in my ears for weeks."

The officer was resilient. "I just need a few days off and I can get back." There was no hesitation in his eyes. I considered asking him if he ever thought about another line of work but didn't. I told him I was going to give him a few more days off. "I think you need a few extra days. You've had a bad year." All he said in reply was, "God bless you."

CHAPTER 14.

THE STANDING DETECTIVE

THE DETECTIVE WOULD NOT SIT DOWN. HE WAS ONE OF SEVERAL members of the service that have come into my office and remained standing throughout the visit. "I'm in a lot of pain," he explained. "And sitting makes it worse."

I've seen a large number of officers with bad backs in my time as a police surgeon; so many that I've come to believe that it is an occupational hazard for members of the department. Perhaps it is the long hours police officers spend on their feet, or behind the wheel of an RMP, or the weight of the gun belt that uniformed officers wear that contributes to this common problem. I only know that a day does not go by in my district without my seeing several officers who are out sick because of a back injury. An aching back is also a frequent complaint for the general population and it is not unusual for officers to develop back injuries off duty as well as on.

I asked the standing Detective to tell me what had happened and he said that he had noted stiffness and soreness of his lower back for a few days, but that severe pain had developed on a "Buy and Bust." "This perp was dealing drugs and when we went to arrest him he took off. I started chasing him, but then it hit me. It was like an explosion in my lower back. I went down to my knees. I've had pain before, but nothing like this," he said. His fellow officers called EMS and the Detective was taken to a local emergency room. He continued. "They gave me a shot of morphine and some Valium and sent me home when the pain eased up, but after a few hours it came back."

I had the Detective lift his shirt so I could inspect his lower back and when he did I saw that his lower spine was shifted to one side. Tense muscles had pulled his spine in the direction of the muscle spasm. I palpated the lower back area and found hard, knotted muscles. "Can you try to touch your toes?" I asked, trying to better assess his injury. The officer grimaced and said, "I can't go any farther than this... it hurts too much." As I watched I saw that he could not bend forward at all. He just tensed his already spastic muscles and lowered his head. I asked him if he felt the pain anywhere else. "The pain goes into my buttock and down my left leg," he replied. I knew this to be a sign of nerve irritation that is commonly called *sciatica* (the sciatic nerve emerges between the lower vertebrae of the spine and travels down the leg). He added, "My foot is asleep half the time."

I told the Detective that his pain and numbness could also be a sign of a "slipped" or herniated disk. The disk is a spongy material that sits between each vertebrae of the spine. If it bulges or moves out of its normal location it can press against the nerves that emerge from the spinal cord, producing severe pain.

I also told the officer that I knew exactly what he was experiencing, since I had had three herniated disks myself. As a fellow back sufferer I could empathize with members of the department that reported with an aching back. The Detective asked me how I made out and I knew what he was curious about. "I didn't need surgery," I said. "Just physical therapy." "Surgery is a last resort," I added, since I knew that cops often compare horror stories while they are waiting to be seen and it was not unusual for an officer to come in and tell me that he was just talking to someone with a bad back who "got worse after surgery."

I authorized the Detective to see an orthopedist that would examine him and make recommendations. The officer returned a few days later with a request from the physician for physical therapy and an MRI of the lower spine. I felt both were appropriate and issued the authorizations.

I saw the Detective again two weeks later. He walked in freely without any sign of pain. "I'm feeling a lot better since I started physical therapy," he said. The MRI had shown a bulging disk in his lower back. He would not need surgery—just physical therapy. "My pain is much less now and I can do a lot more," he said. "I know," I replied. "You just sat down."

CHAPTER 15.

THE SERGEANT WITH A TWISTED FACE

POLICE OFFICERS ARE GENERALLY YOUNG AND MALE AND THE ILL-nesses that afflict them commonly strike men between the ages of 20 and 50. Women make up 18 percent of the force, so NYPD surgeons must also be prepared to see officers with gynecological problems. The NYPD has a "pregnancy district" staffed by an obstetrician, who monitors the care of female officers during their pregnancies.

Although most illnesses fit the demographic of these groups based on age and sex, there have been times that I felt that the number or types of illnesses were unusual. An example presented itself in the form of an officer I saw who awoke and found that the left side of his face was "crooked." He was unable to close his left eye and when he tried to smile he could not lift the left side of his mouth. "I look like I've had a stroke, "he said. The officer saw his primary physician who diagnosed "Bell's palsy." This condition results from paralysis of the facial nerve and has no known cause. Most physicians feel that it results from a viral infection.

The officer in question was fitted with an eye patch and placed on antiviral medication and corticosteroids, the time--honored medical approach to this problem. He had finished these medications by the time I saw him in the district, but had not improved. I was amazed to see this officer because I had just seen a female sergeant with facial paralysis and could think of at least four or five other cases that I had seen in my district in what I thought was a relatively short time. I wondered if there was a common source. The sergeant in fact had a much more severe illness that produced headache and other neurological signs. The source of her illness was found to be Lyme disease that had spread into her nervous system.

My district is made up of area codes that cover the north Bronx and northern suburbs of New York City. These are often wooded areas that are prime real estate for the tick that causes Lyme disease. I wondered if this might explain why I was seeing more cases of Bell's palsy. I found that the medical literature had noticed this association as well, and that at least one article I read called for the treatment of Lyme disease in all cases of Bell's Palsy. I now ask all of the officers I see with this condition if they have been tested for Lyme.

I saw the Sergeant several times in my district office while she was receiving antibiotics for her infection. "I still have headaches, some dizziness, but I feel that the treatment is working," she said. I looked at her face on her second visit and found that it looked perfectly normal. She noticed my gaze and said, "It's gone, or mostly gone. I think I can detect a little droop of the corner of my mouth, but no one else can see it. It's so good to be able to close my eye."

I asked her if she remembered any tick bites. "No, not one. That's the strangest thing, although everyone tells me that it is not unusual to miss the bite. I wasn't feeling great for a few weeks, but I would never have guessed it was Lyme disease. I just got up one morning with my face all twisted and a pounding headache."

The Sergeant returned after finishing three weeks of therapy and I asked if she was ready to return to work. Her reply was an emphatic: "Yes!" I must have looked surprised because she began to explain that the weeks of confinement had been difficult. "I've been in my house for a long time. Even when I wasn't receiving the intravenous I avoided going out in our backyard for fear of another bite. I can't wait to get back. Manhattan will look like paradise to me. I don't want to see green."

CHAPTER 16.

WEEKEND SICK

I HEARD THE NEXT OFFICER TO BE SEEN ONE SUNDAY MORNING BE-
fore he came into view. It was my turn to take weekend sick call. In my
time as a police surgeon I've developed an ear for the sounds a person
makes when they are using crutches. There's a rhythmic thump of the
crutch followed by the sweeping noise of the good leg. As the officer came
down the hallway towards my office I thought, "Knee or ankle?"

It was a knee, as the large immobilizer strapped around the young
man's left leg told me. I asked him to tell me what happened. "I had this
dealer under surveillance and then he saw me and took off. I chased him
for several blocks and then I jumped over some trash. When I landed I
turned and I think I heard a 'pop.' My knee just gave out from under me."

The officer was taken to the ER, where x--rays were taken. He continued. "They said nothing's broken but they think from the exam that it's
my ACL (anterior cruciate ligament). I got strapped into this brace and
they said not to put any weight on it, but I tried walking and it gave out
again." I authorized a consultation with an orthopedist who I knew would
certainly request an MRI.

The ACL is one of four major ligaments that stabilize the knee. If the
scan confirmed an ACL tear the officer would need to have surgery and
undergo extensive rehabilitation. Although the majority of these injuries

are successfully treated, an ACL tear may be a career--ending injury. I could not predict what the future held for this particular officer. All I could do was wish him luck and ask him to send in the next person in line.

I see injured officers at my district office on weekdays. On weekends and holidays the medical offices are closed, so any officer reporting sick must report to medical headquarters in Queens. The police surgeon on call for these days sees all of the officers who are out sick and then takes call until the next morning, travelling to hospitals when a member of the service is admitted.

On this particular Sunday morning about 50 officers were gathered waiting to see me with a wide variety of complaints and illnesses. I often think of these tours as my "MASH" experience, since I need to quickly assess what's wrong and how severely ill each individual is, as well as when the officer may return to work.

I did a double take when I saw the young female office sit down. Her right eye was badly blackened and her jaw was swollen. I noticed bruises on both her hands and arms. I didn't have to ask her to tell me her story; she started when she saw me staring at her face. "There was this group of girls harassing people on the street. They looked like gang members. As soon as I approached them they attacked me, punching and pulling my hair. My partner tried to mace them but I ended up getting more than they did. I got popped pretty good."

I asked her if x--rays had been done in the ER, since I had seen a few officers with fractures of the bony orbit that supports the eye. "Yeah, they x--rayed and I even had a CAT scan, since I hit my head on the pavement. I'm just black and blue and I have a bad headache."

I tried to remember when I had last seen a woman with this type of injury and could only think of a battered wife that had come to the ER when I was still an Intern. Although the circumstances were much different, I was still disturbed by the officer's appearance. Prior to joining the department I had never thought of female police officers as being exposed to the same dangers as their male counterparts. But there was no room for a weaker sex in the Department. She must have sensed my alarm since she

said, "This will get better. I'm not worried. It comes with the territory."
I told her to rest for a week and then come back for me to see if she was
ready to return to duty. She seemed relieved to have the time off.

I finished my tour and headed home to await any trauma calls. None
came, but I slept fitfully expecting to be called out. The disturbing image
of the battered female officer drifted in and out of my mind. In my sleep I
saw that the territory she spoke of was a dangerous place.

CHAPTER 17.

ASSAULTED

I HAD NOT THOUGHT OF POLICE OFFICERS AS VICTIMS OF VIOLENT crime until I met a young officer at my district office. She walked in without any visible signs of trauma. Her demeanor gave me the impression that she did not want to be here and did not suggest that she was injured. I asked her to tell me what brought her and she made eye contact and said, "I was raped."

Her response was so unexpected that I knew that my expression must have shown surprise. I could detect no emotion on her part. Officers had reported to me with every type of injury, but this was the first time I had seen one for sexual assault. I asked her if she minded telling me what happened and she replied, "It was a stalker."

I noticed an edge in her voice as she continued, "I had an order of protection. He's made advances and threats before and followed me. Two nights ago I was coming home and he must have been waiting. I got my key in the door and he forced me from behind.

"Then he attacked me."

She told me she had reported the assault and that her attacker was being held. I asked if she had seen a rape counselor. There were no tears, only the edge in her voice that nearly broke. "Yes," she replied. "I'm okay." I suspected that she was far from being all right and asked if she was sleeping.

She said, "I've had some bad nights." I suggested that she see call her coun-selor and she said she would.

Then she added, "Staying home is killing me, I want to get back to work." I told her I was concerned about how recent the attack had been and her lack of sleep clouding her judgment. She added, "But I can't be home. I'd feel better at work." I realized that she wanted to be away from where the attack had taken place. We decided on her returning to light duty in a few days. I saw her one more time a few weeks later when she again reassured me that she was well. I returned her to full duty still un-able to see much beyond her exterior.

A few months later I saw two officers in one morning who were vi-ciously attacked in an area in Brooklyn, possibly by the same perpetrator.

The first was a young Hispanic officer who said that he had been "sucker punched" as he walked down a street. The officer was startled by the blow and felt severe pain in his jaw, but then saw a stream of blood coming from his face. He was taken to an emergency room where he was told that his attacker must have had a razor since he had a large gash from under his right eye to near the corner of his mouth. The officer removed his bandage for me to see. I wondered if his laceration would leave a prom-inent scar. The officer must have read my mind, since he asked if I thought he'd have a bad scar. I told him that it was hard to predict at this time but that dermatologists were treating scars with lasers and that I could refer him to someone I knew. I suggested that he see a plastic surgeon now and he agreed. I also asked him about his attacker, who had fled and not been apprehended. "I don't know much; just that he must be disturbed, and hate cops."

Three individuals attacked the second officer as he patrolled on foot in the same area. One of the men wrestled with the officer and succeeded in taking his gun, using it to pound his head and face repeatedly. The of-ficer was taken to an emergency room where CAT scans showed small fractures of the skull and facial bones. The officer had one laceration near the hairline and another near his mouth. His face appeared swollen, but he had no trouble speaking and I thought that he looked surprisingly upbeat for someone who had been so violently beaten. I asked if his attackers had been caught and his expression darkened. "No, not yet." I wasn't sure if his reaction was due to frustration that his attackers were free or fear that he could be a target again. I told him that because of the fractures he would not be able to return to duty for a few weeks. The officer tried to grin and said, "Maybe they'll be locked up by the time I get back."

As my time as a police surgeon has grown I've shed the illusion that officers of the law are somehow immune from the maladies that afflict all men and women in our society. They have the same number of accidents, illnesses, and tragedies of fate that befall us all. They may protect us from crime and uphold the rule of law, but they too may be victims.

CHAPTER 18.

FIT FOR DUTY

I TRIED TO IMAGINE WHAT THE OFFICER WAS DESCRIBING AS WE sat in my district office. Every day I hear descriptions of how members of the service are injured, and some are vivid descriptions that stay in my mind. The officer, a sixteen-year veteran of the force, was assigned to Robbery and he and his partner were following a suspect in a number of burglaries that had occurred in the last few months. He said that such surveillance often didn't produce results but on this occasion they had hit pay dirt.

"We saw our guy meet someone and then the two of them drove into Queens. They stopped and went around the side of a house. After about 20 minutes we followed them and when I got to the house I looked in a window and saw someone duck taped to a chair. It looked like a home invasion."

The officer went on to describe how he and his partner entered the home and encountered the two suspects loading property into a garbage bag. "They were surprised to see us but they made it clear that they were going to fight and would not cooperate. They had the owner of the home tied and taped and he looked like he had been beaten."

A struggle ensued with the two officers paired off with the suspects in hand-to-hand combat. My cop got punched, kicked, and thrown to the floor, but managed to subdue his assailant. He ended up helping his partner fight off the other suspect, who he described as "large." "They were pretty tough," he said with a painful grin since he had been hit in the mouth.

I looked at the officer emergency room discharge sheet that listed his injuries: contusions both hands, arms, face, knees, sprain of the shoulder, neck, mid-, and lower-back and said. "I'd say you were tougher."

The officer smiled as best he could. He said the best part was untying the homeowner, who thanked the police officers profusely. "He was pretty happy to see us." I could see that the officer felt good about his arrest. At that moment the struggle with the two perpetrators and the pain of his injuries must have seemed insignificant, since he said, "When can I get back to work? I don't want to be at a desk. Put me back full duty."

I told him I admired his dedication but that I couldn't put him back until I was sure he was up to it. "I don't have to tell you what you might run into on the street," I said. "Just imagine that you ran into these two *large* guys today, in your condition." The officer reluctantly agreed to some time off to allow his injuries to heal. He would return to me in a week and, if he was improved, then return to work.

The officer's request to return to full duty while still injured is not an uncommon request for me to deal with. Although I am sympathetic to the desire to return to duty, I have to place the safety of both the officer and the public that they are protecting first. I sensed my Robbery cop's pride and satisfaction at capturing two dangerous criminals. He wanted to get back and pursue other violent individuals. As a citizen I wanted him out there, but as his district surgeon I had to be sure that he was fit for duty.

CHAPTER 19.

WYCKOFF

FROM THE MOMENT I KNEW THAT I WOULD BE VISITING HOSPITALS to see injured police officers I realized that I was certain to be called to visit one particular hospital in Brooklyn that I knew well. I also knew that it would be a difficult trip, not because of the distance or neighborhood that surrounded it, but because it would call up so many memories.

After more than four years on the job the call I was waiting for came on a recent Sunday night, awakening me from much-needed sleep. The sergeant at the Sick Desk apologized for disturbing me and said, "An officer got admitted to Wyckoff…" I did not hear much more but managed to get the officer's name and injury.

"Wyckoff," or "Wyckoff Heights Hospital," is a name I have known since I was a child. The name was part of my vocabulary before I could identify much of my environment. Wyckoff was my Dad's hospital and the place he would go when he left his family each morning, and often during the night, for an emergency. "Wyckoff" was often on the phone, interrupting meals and our time together, taking my father away when I desperately wanted him to stay. As I grew older it was also the place my Dad would take me to begin my medical education. At first I was an observer, watching him make rounds and interact with his patients. Later I was given jobs around the hospital during summer vacations, and before starting medical school I did an externship where I learned the basics of diagnosis and treatment.

But my ties to Wyckoff went even deeper and were formed before I was born. In 1939 my Dad started his internship there. One day he was eating lunch with a colleague and an attractive dark-haired nurse walked by. My Dad was immediately smitten and asked his friend if he knew who she was. "Her name's Rose and she's the head nurse on Male Ward." My father was not satisfied with that — he wanted every detail. In a short time they were dating and they would marry the same year. Following my mother's death I found a photograph among her things of the two of them in crisp white uniforms standing on a fire escape at Wyckoff. In the photo my Dad cannot keep his eyes off of my mother while she smiles toward the camera. Taken before their marriage and the impending struggles of war and family, it captured the essence of their love.

I asked for Highway to take me to see the injured officer at Wyckoff. As we pulled out to go the officer said he had placed the location in his GPS, since he had never been there before. I had made the trip many times but not for more than 15 years. In the darkness I was happy for the guidance. As we got closer, however, I began to see familiar landmarks and street signs and to feel a rush of memories. Wyckoff Heights Hospital is located on the Brooklyn--Queens border in a low--income neighborhood known as Bushwick. I could see that the years had not been kind to the area, and as we reached the hospital I noticed that there had been considerable construction. The Emergency Room entrance was now much larger and did not resemble what I remembered. I began to doubt if the fire escape that my parents stood on more than 70 years earlier still existed.

We passed the ER entrance and turned the corner to discover that the main entrance had been relocated and expanded. I thought about the many times I had entered this building and wondered what I would find. I looked for familiar landmarks and found none – the lobby had been entirely reconstructed. I had to ask for directions to reach the injured officer's room.

The officer was a young woman who had developed sudden dizziness and arm weakness. She had a history of severe high blood pressure and a previous stroke. She was comfortable when I found her and said that her symptoms had resolved. I spoke with the physicians who had attended her and found that an MRI of the brain had been ordered. If the results were favorable she would most likely be discharged in the morning.

My duties at Wyckoff were done but I could not help lingering in the lobby, where I found a memorial to physicians who had distinguished themselves as members of the staff. I recognized many of the names as colleagues of my father's and remembered how he had introduced me to each one on my first day of work there. I left the hospital reluctantly, still hoping to see something that would connect me with the past. Highway pulled away and as we approached the next corner I saw part of the old Wyckoff Hospital come into view, a jet-- black building that had always reminded me of a medieval castle. We stopped for a red light and there, in the darkness on the second floor, I saw the fire escape that my parents had stood on. I thought about that moment when they had posed together and the love that sustained them for fifty-five years.

The light changed and we moved on.

CHAPTER 20.

OCCUPIED

I BEGAN TO SEE INJURIES THAT OCCURRED AT THE OCCUPY WALL
Street demonstrations about a month after the protest started. They were
not major injuries; most of them were bruises and small lacerations from
trying to handcuff individuals who were resisting arrest.

I had watched the news coverage and some of the YouTube videos,
which showed police officers accused of using excessive force. One officer
told me that he had three friends in the department who were on YouTube
and that all of them felt that they had been unfairly portrayed. As a member of the service I felt sympathy for the police officers who were placed
under the scrutiny of the video camera during highly stressful situations.

I asked several officers who reported sick what it was like during their
details downtown and the most common response was that they were
bored. One officer said, "It's a lot of standing around, watching and listening to them, and not much else to do." I got the impression that there had
been an order to restrain from confrontation with the demonstrators and
that most had complied. They had also been trained to arrest anyone who
broke the law or resisted.

There seemed to be considerable distain among members of the service for the group encamped at Zuccotti Park. One officer said, "They
think it's Woodstock and the '60s' all over again and a lot of homeless have

joined them. I wouldn't want to spend the night there myself. I heard that there was an outbreak of scabies. They're having sex and drug parties."

After a month of demonstrations and encampment I noticed that the nature of the injuries the officers experienced downtown appeared to change. Some of the injuries were more severe and one of the officers said that the demonstrators seemed more inclined to fight. "No one's going peacefully," he said. The atmosphere had become more intense as well. "They're in your face, telling you that you are a fascist, a capitalist tool, a pig, you name it. They're throwing things, even feces; you have to keep your head down."

One officer seemed particularly upset. "I'm all for civil disobedience. I believe in it. Before I became a police officer I did my share for civil rights. I was on a lot of marches and I never got arrested. Now I'm on the other side of the barricades and it's hard; I'm sympathetic, but if anyone throws anything at me, he's going to the hospital!"

As a group, the officers seemed impatient with the mayor as the encampment continued. "It's time for these people to go. It smells, it's noisy, what are they waiting for?" said one frustrated cop. I saw a few officers for injuries they sustained in the operation to clear the park. Most had been injured in direct hand-to-hand combat with demonstrators. Although battered, all of them were happy the occupation was over. "I'm for free speech," one of them said, "but I don't think they should ever have been allowed to camp out. Enough is enough; it was time for them to go."

I saw the same officer a week later and asked how things stood now. "They can't camp out, but they can stand or sit there all night. There's a group of about a hundred or so during the day. It's gotten colder and it's hard to keep warm when you're standing on your feet all night. The churches are letting them sleep over but a few diehards are sitting outside and we still got to watch."

I said that I thought that a lot of other cities had not done as well as we had in handling the same situation and he smiled a big grin. "Yeah, I saw that. Look at Philadelphia and Oakland. It took them longer than we did and a lot more people got hurt. We were lucky that it got cold, but I think they will be back in the spring. That means we'll be back too."

CHAPTER 21.

BE WELL AND STAY SAFE

MY FIVE-YEAR ANNIVERSARY WITH THE NYPD PASSED IN DECEMBER 2011 and I remain on the job, second in seniority at my district in the Bronx and fifteenth overall among my fellow surgeons. Seniority is important in the NYPD, since it affects assignments and vacation picks. I was fortunate that a few police surgeons were hired not long after I joined the force, so I wasn't last on the seniority list very long. Last means that you have little choice but to accept what is left after everyone else has chosen.

After more than 30 years in practice I did not expect that I would learn a lot as a police surgeon but in fact the variety of injuries and illnesses has taught me a great deal. I believe that by the time I reach my goal of 20 years of service I will have seen an injury to every joint or bone in the human body. At the same time I continue to see common medical problems like obesity, producing diabetes, hypertension, and sleep apnea in a growing number of members of the service. This has produced a new reason for officers to report sick — gastric bypass surgery. Problems such as kidney stones, diverticulitis, gout, as well as elective surgeries such as vasectomy, deviated septum, and liposuction continue to cross my desk.

The psychological effects of violence directed at members of the service remains a common problem. One of my officers, who was assaulted on the job, developed post-traumatic stress disorder. Her frequent flash backs and nightmares were as disabling as her physical injuries. At this time she has benefited greatly from seeing one of the NYPD's psychiatrists and is about to resume full duty.

I do not see as many members of the service who were injured on 9/11 since many have retired; it is less common for me to be asked to evaluate the records of an officer who has applied for disability retirement based on lung disease. The Department continues to monitor the lung function of first responders who choose to be tested and has published these results, as has the FDNY. Further monitoring will also focus on whether there is an increase in the number of malignancies in this group.

I've shortened my daily trek to the 50th Precinct by learning more than one alternate route that takes me to and from midtown Manhattan along side streets that are usually less crowded. Traffic jams are still common, but I've come to accept the fact that I may have to sit in traffic. I keep looking for new shortcuts and have several smartphone traffic apps complete with camera views that tell me where the bottlenecks are.

Trauma calls have varied from all night visits to multiple hospitals to relatively calm nights, but I find that I still sleep fitfully whenever I am on call. Major traumas to members of the service have continued to occur, both on and off duty, with more shootings in past few months. Sadly, the increased violence directed at police officers appears to be a national trend. I was thankful that the last officer I saw at Bellevue who was shot was "not likely."

Many of the officers I see know me from previous "sicks" and ask about my family when they come in. A number have seen the pictures of my dogs on the bulletin board in my office and want to talk about their pets. A few have listened to my weekly show on SiriusXM and may comment on what they heard. In this way my work as a police surgeon is not much different from my medical practice — the relationships formed may be just as strong, even though my primary role as a police surgeon is to assess the fitness for duty of these men and women and not to provide care.

The five-year anniversary brought some pay benefits, but above all I enjoy my work with the NYPD. I respect what police officers instinctively do to protect the public, typically with complete disregard of their own wellbeing. This has made me an unabashed supporter of the NYPD, despite occasional headlines that shout "bad cop."

Police surgeons are not popular members of the department since the decision to return someone to work is not always welcomed. Most of the time, however, it is and every day I see members of the service who enthusiastically say, "Put me back — full duty." I personally relish seeing an injured officer returned to good health and able to resume his work. My five years with the NYPD has made me acutely aware of the dangers and potential injuries that these individuals may face. I would like to protect them all from harm but all I can do is hope that they will be well and stay safe.

APPENDIX

NYPD FACTS

Founded	1844
Uniformed Members	34,500
Budget	$3.9 Billion
Headquarters	One Police Plaza
Nickname	*New York's Finest*
Motto	*Fidelis ad Mortem*
	Faithful Unto Death
Jurisdiction	City of New York (Population 8,175,133)
Commands	76 Precincts
	12 Transit Districts
	9 Housing Police Service Areas
Police Cars	8,839
Police Boats	11
Helicopters	8

Horses	120
Dogs	31 German Shepherds 3 Bloodhounds
Website	http//:www.nyc.gov/html/nypd/

NYPD RANKS (descending order)

Chief of Department

Bureau Chief

Assistant Chief

Deputy Chief

Inspector

Deputy Inspector

Captain

Lieutenant

Sergeant

Detective (grades 1-3)

Police Officer

Probationary Police Officer

Cadet

COMMISSIONER TITLES

Police Commissioner

First Deputy Commissioner

Deputy Commissioner

COMMON NYPD RADIO CODES

10-1	Call Your Command
10-2	Return to Your Command
10-3	Call Dispatcher by Telephone
10-4	Acknowledgement
10-5	Repeat Message
10-6	Standby
10-7	Verify Address
10-10	Possible Crime (prowler suspicious person/vehicle, shots fired, etc.)
10-11	Alarm
10-12	Police Officer/Security Holding Suspect
10-13	Assist Police Officer
10-14	License Plate Check – Occupied & Suspicious – Verify If Stolen
10-15	License Plate Check – Verify If Stolen – Occupied or Not
10-16	Vehicle is Reported Stolen
10-17	Vehicle is Not Reported Stolen
10-18	Warrant Check Shows an Active Warrant
10-19	Warrant Check Negative
10-20/10-30	Robbery/Burglary/Larceny (Past/Crime-In Progress)
10-21/10-31	Explosive Device or Threat
10-22/10-32	Assault/Child Abuse
10-50	Disorderly Person/Group or Noise
10-53	Vehicle Accident
10-63	Out of Service – Meal

10-66	Unusual Incident (train derailment/collision, plane crash, building collapse)
10-75	Vertical Patrol
10-85	Need Additional Unit
10-92	Arrest
10-98	Resuming patrol/available

www.ingramcontent.com/pod-product-compliance
Lightning Source LLC
Chambersburg PA
CBHW021239280526
45784CB00005B/2157